Keto Vegetarian Delicacies

Flavorful Low-Carb Vegetarian
Recipes for a Balanced Healthy Diet

Ricardo Abagnale

o

By reading this document, the reader agrees that under no circumstances is the author responsible for any losses, direct or indirect, which are incurred as a result of the use of information contained within this document, including, but not limited to, — errors, omissions, or inaccuracies.

Table of Contents

4

INTRODUCTION

The Ketogenic diet is truly life changing. The diet improves your overall health and helps you lose the extra weight in a matter of days. The diet will show its multiple benefits even from the beginning and it will become your new lifestyle really soon.

As soon as you embrace the Ketogenic diet, you will start to live a completely new life.

On the other hand, the vegetarian diet is such a healthy dietary option you can choose when trying to live healthy and also lose some weight.

The collection we bring to you today is actually a combination between the Ketogenic and vegetarian diets. You get to discover some amazing Ketogenic vegetarian dishes you can prepare in the comfort of your own home. All the dishes you found here follow both the Ketogenic and the vegetarian rules, they all taste delicious and rich and they are all easy to make.

We can assure you that such a combo is hard to find. So, start a keto diet with a vegetarian "touch" today. It will be both useful and fun!

So, what are you still waiting for? Get started with the Ketogenic diet and learn how to prepare the best and most flavored Ketogenic vegetarian dishes. Enjoy them all!

Vanilla Chia Breakfast Pudding

Preparation time: 10 minutes

Servings: 2

Nutritional Values (Per Serving):

- Calories: 223
- Fat: 12 g
- Carbohydrates: 18 g
- Sugar: 2 g
- Protein: 10 g
- Cholesterol: 0 mg

Ingredients:

- ½ cup blueberries for topping
- 6 tablespoons chia seeds
- 2 cups coconut milk, unsweetened
- ½ teaspoon vanilla extract

Directions:

1. Add the coconut milk, chia seeds, vanilla to a glass jar. Seal the jar and shake well. Place the jar in the fridge overnight.
2. The next morning, pour the chia breakfast pudding into serving bowls and top with blueberries.
3. Serve and enjoy!

Almond Cinnamon Smoothie

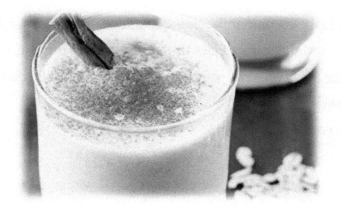

Preparation time: 10 minutes

Servings: 1

Nutritional Values (Per Serving):

- Calories: 500
- Fat: 43 g
- Carbohydrates: 10 g
- Sugar: 2 g
- Protein: 14.6 g
- Cholesterol: 0 mg

Ingredients:

- ¾ cup almond milk, unsweetened

- ¼ cup coconut oil
- 1 tablespoon almond butter, unsweetened
- 1 tablespoon vanilla protein powder
- 1/8 teaspoon cinnamon

Directions:

1. Add into your blender all the ingredients, blend them until they are nice and smooth.
2. Serve and enjoy!

Mashed Turnips

Preparation time: 5 minutes

Cooking time: 20 minutes

Servings: 4

Nutritional Values (Per Serving):

- Calories: 132
- Cholesterol: 33 mg
- Protein: 1.2 g
- Carbohydrates: 7 g
- Fat: 11.5 g

Ingredients:

- 3 cups turnip, diced
- 2 garlic cloves, minced
- ¼ cup heavy cream

- 3 tablespoons butter, melted
- Pepper and salt to taste

Directions:

1. Bring your turnip to a boil in a saucepan over medium heat. Cook for about 20 minutes, then drain turnips and mash until smooth.
2. Add butter, garlic, heavy cream, pepper, and salt. Mix well.
3. Serve warm and enjoy!

Creamy Coconut Curry

Preparation time: 15 minutes

Cooking time: 30 minutes

Servings: 4

Nutritional Values (Per Serving):

- Calories: 235
- Cholesterol: 0 mg
- Sugar: 2.1 g
- Carbohydrates: 8.4 g
- Fat: 22.3 g
- Protein: 4.1 g

Ingredients:

- 1 teaspoon garlic, minced
- 1 teaspoon ginger, minced
- 2 teaspoons soy sauce
- 1 tablespoon red curry paste

- 1 cup broccoli florets
- 1 handful spinach
- ¼ of an onion, sliced
- ½ cup coconut cream
- 4 tablespoons coconut oil

Directions:

1. In a saucepan over medium-high heat, heat your coconut oil.
2. Add your onion to the pan and cook until softened. Add garlic and cook until lightly browned.
3. Reduce heat to medium-low, adding broccoli, stir well. Cook for about 20 minutes then add the curry paste and stir. Add spinach over broccoli and cook until wilted.
4. Add soy sauce, ginger and coconut cream, and stir. Simmer for an additional 10 minutes. Serve hot and enjoy!

Broccoli Omelet

Preparation time: 10 minutes

Cooking time: 10 minutes

Servings: 2

Nutritional Values (Per Serving):

- Calories: 203
- Fat: 15.9 g
- Cholesterol: 327 mg
- Protein: 12.4 g
- Carbohydrates: 4 g
- Sugar: 1.5 g

Ingredients:

- 1 tablespoon extra-virgin olive oil
- 1 tablespoon parsley, chopped
- 1 cup broccoli, cooked, chopped
- 4 eggs, organic

- ½ teaspoon sea salt
- ¼ teaspoon pepper

Directions:

1. In a mixing bowl beat eggs with salt and pepper. Add broccoli to egg mixture.
2. Heat the olive oil in a pan over medium heat. Pour your broccoli and eggs mixture into the pan and cook until set. Flip and cook other side until lightly browned.
3. Garnish with chopped parsley. Serve and joy!

Tomato Soup

Preparation time: 10 minutes

Cooking time: 20 minutes

Servings: 4

Nutritional Values (Per Serving):

- Calories: 125
- Cholesterol: 0 mg
- Protein: 7.2 g
- Sugar: 8 g
- Carbohydrates:
- 13.7 g
- Fat: 5.4 g

Ingredients:

- 2 tablespoons tomato paste
- 1 tablespoon garlic, minced
- 1 tablespoon extra-virgin olive oil

- 4 cups vegetable broth, low-sodium
- ½ teaspoon thyme, chopped, fresh
- 1 tablespoon basil, fresh, chopped
- 1 teaspoon oregano, fresh, chopped
- 1 cup onion, chopped
- 1 cup red bell pepper, chopped
- 3 cups tomatoes, peeled, seeded, chopped
- ¼ teaspoon pepper

Directions:

1. In the saucepan heat your oil over medium heat.
2. Add bell pepper, garlic, onion, and tomatoes, sauté for 10 minutes. Add remaining ingredients and stir to combine. Increase the heat to high and bring to a boil. Reduce heat to low and place a lid on the pan and simmer for 10 minutes. Remove from heat.
3. Puree the soup using a blender until smooth.
4. Serve and enjoy!

Tofu Scramble

Preparation time: 10 minutes **Cooking time:** 10 minutes
Servings: 4

Nutritional Values (Per Serving):

- Calories: 105
- Cholesterol: 0mg
- Sugar: 3.7 g
- Fat: 5 g
- Carbohydrates: 7.6 g
- Protein: 10.6 g

Ingredients:

- 1 garlic clove, minced
- 1 cup mushrooms, sliced
- ½ teaspoon turmeric
- ½ teaspoon pepper
- ½ teaspoon sea salt
- 1 small onion, diced

- 1 tomato, diced
- 1 bell pepper, diced
- 1 lb. tofu, firm, drained

Directions:

1. Heat a pan over medium heat, adding mushrooms, tomato, onion, garlic and bell pepper, sauté veggies for 5 minutes.
2. Crumble the tofu into pan over the veggies. Add pepper, turmeric, sea salt and stir well. Cook tofu for 5 minutes.
3. Serve and enjoy!

Mashed Cauliflower

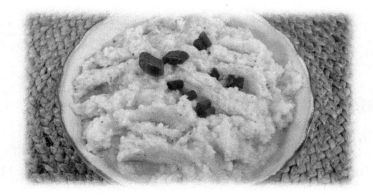

Preparation time: 10 minutes

Cooking time: 15 minutes

Servings: 6

Nutritional Values (Per Serving):

- Calories: 120
- Fat: 8 g
- Cholesterol: 21 mg
- Sugar: 5 g
- Carbohydrates: 10.9 g
- Protein: 4.1 g

Ingredients:

- 2 tablespoons milk
- 4 tablespoons butter
- 2 cauliflower heads, cut into florets
- ½ teaspoon onion powder
- ½ teaspoon garlic powder
- ½ teaspoon sea salt
- ½ teaspoon pepper

Directions:

1. Add your cauliflower to a saucepan filled with enough water to cover the cauliflower. Cook cauliflower over medium heat for 15 minutes.
2. Drain your cauliflower florets and place it in a mixing bowl. Add remaining ingredients to the bowl.
3. Using a blender blend until smooth. Serve and enjoy!

Roasted Cauliflower

Preparation time: 10 minutes

Cooking time: 30 minutes

Servings: 4

Nutritional Values (Per Serving):

- Calories: 87
- Cholesterol: 0 mg
- Sugar: 5.1 g
- Carbohydrates: 12 g
- Fat: 3.8 g
- Protein: 4.3 g

Ingredients:

- 1 cauliflower head, cut into florets
- 2 tablespoons fresh sage, chopped
- 1 garlic clove, minced
- 1 tablespoon extra-virgin olive oil

Directions:

1. Preheat your oven to 400°Fahrenheit. Coat a baking tray with cooking spray. Spread the cauliflower florets on prepared baking tray. Bake cauliflower in the oven for 30 minutes.

2. Meanwhile, sauté garlic in a pan with one tablespoon of olive oil. Remove from heat and set aside.

3. Add cauliflower, garlic, and sage to a bowl and toss to mix.

4. Serve and enjoy!

Roasted Green Beans

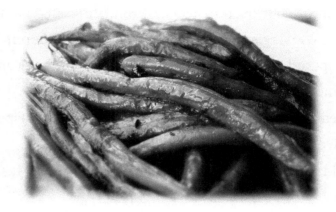

Preparation time: 15 minutes

Cooking time: 30 minutes

Servings: 4

Nutritional Values (Per Serving):

Calories: 98

Sugar: 1.8 g

Carbohydrates: 8.8 g

Fat: 7.2 g

Cholesterol: 0 mg

Protein: 2.2 g

Ingredients:

- 1 lb. green beans, frozen
- 2 tablespoons extra-virgin olive oil
- ½ teaspoon onion powder
- ½ teaspoon garlic powder
- ½ teaspoon sea salt
- ½ teaspoon pepper

Directions:

1. Preheat your oven to 425°Fahrenheit. Spray a cooking tray with cooking spray.
2. In a bowl add all your ingredients and mix well. Spread the green beans on the prepared baking tray and bake for 30 minutes.
3. Serve and enjoy!

Creamy Cauliflower Spinach Soup

Preparation time: 10 minutes

Cooking time: 35 minutes

Servings: 5

Nutritional Values (Per Serving):

- Calories: 153
- Cholesterol: 0 mg
- Sugar: 4.3 g
- Fat: 8.3 g
- Carbohydrates: 8.7 g
- Protein: 11.9 g

Ingredients:

- 5 watercress, chopped
- 8 cups vegetable broth
- 1 lb. cauliflower, chopped
- 5-ounces spinach, fresh, chopped

- ½ cup coconut milk
- Sea salt

Directions:

1. Add cauliflower along with broth to a large pot over medium heat for 15 minutes, bring to a boil. Add spinach and watercress, cook for another 10 minutes.
2. Remove from heat and using a blender puree the soup until smooth.
3. Add coconut milk and stir well. Season with sea salt.
4. Serve hot and enjoy!

Tomato Quinoa

Preparation time: 10 minutes

Cooking time: 25 minutes

Servings: 4

Nutritional Values (Per Serving):

- Calories 202
- Fat 4
- Fiber 2
- Carbs 12
- Protein 10

Ingredients:

- 1 cup quinoa
- 3 cups chicken stock
- 1 cup tomatoes, cubed
- 1 tablespoon parsley, chopped

- 1 tablespoon basil, chopped
- 1 teaspoon turmeric powder
- A pinch of salt and black pepper

Directions:

1. In a pot, mix the quinoa with the stock, the tomatoes and the other ingredients, toss, bring to a simmer and cook over medium heat for 25 minutes.
2. Divide everything between plates and serve.

Coriander Black Beans

Preparation time: 10 minutes

Cooking time: 20 minutes

Servings: 4

Nutritional Values (Per Serving):

- Calories 221
- Fat 5
- Fiber 4
- Carbs 9
- Protein 11

Ingredients:

- 1 tablespoon olive oil
- 2 cups canned black beans, drained and rinsed
- 1 green bell pepper, chopped
- 1 yellow onion, chopped
- 4 garlic cloves, minced

- 1 teaspoon cumin, ground
- ½ cup chicken stock
- 1 tablespoon coriander, chopped
- A pinch of salt and black pepper

Directions:

1. Heat up a pan with the oil over medium heat, add the onion and the garlic and sauté for 5 minutes.
2. Add the black beans and the other ingredients, toss, cook over medium heat for 15 minutes more, divide between plates and serve.

Green Beans and Mango Mix

Preparation time: 10 minutes

Cooking time: 20 minutes

Servings: 4

Nutritional Values (Per Serving):

- Calories 182
- Fat 4
- Fiber 5
- Carbs 6
- Protein 8

Ingredients:

- 1 pound green beans, trimmed and halved
- 3 scallions, chopped
- 1 mango, peeled and cubed
- 2 tablespoons olive oil
- ½ cup veggie stock

- 1 tablespoon oregano, chopped
- 1 teaspoon sweet paprika
- A pinch of salt and black pepper

Directions:

1. Heat up a pan with the oil over medium heat, add the scallions and sauté for 2 minutes.
2. Add the green beans and the other ingredients, toss, cook over medium heat for 18 minutes more, divide between plates and serve.

Quinoa with Olives

Preparation time: 10 minutes

Cooking time: 30 minutes

Servings: 4

Nutritional Values (Per Serving):

- Calories 261
- Fat 6
- Fiber 8
- Carbs 10
- Protein 6

Ingredients:

- 1 yellow onion, chopped
- 1 tablespoon olive oil
- 1 cup quinoa
- 3 cups vegetable stock
- ½ cup black olives, pitted and halved

- 2 green onions, chopped
- 2 tablespoons coconut aminos
- 1 teaspoon rosemary, dried

Directions:

1. Heat up a pot with the oil over medium heat, add the yellow onion and sauté for 5 minutes.
2. Add the quinoa and the other ingredients except the green onions, stir, bring to a simmer and cook over medium heat for 25 minutes.
3. Divide the mix between plates, sprinkle the green onions on top and serve.

Sweet Potato Mash

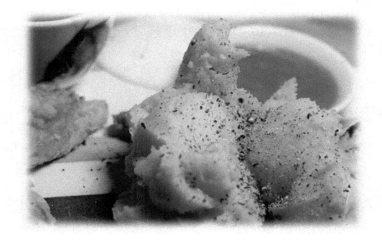

Preparation time: 10 minutes

Cooking time: 25 minutes

Servings: 4

Nutritional Values (Per Serving):

- Calories 200
- Fat 4
- Fiber 4
- Carbs 7
- Protein 10

Ingredients:

- 1 cup veggie stock
- 1 pound sweet potatoes, peeled and cubed
- 1 cup coconut cream
- 2 teaspoons olive oil
- A pinch of salt and black pepper
- ½ teaspoon turmeric powder
- 1 tablespoon chives, chopped

Directions:

1. In a pot, combine the stock with the sweet potatoes and the other ingredients except the cream, the oil and the chives, stir, bring to a simmer and cook over medium heat fro 25 minutes.
2. Add the rest of the ingredients, mash the mix well, stir it, divide between plates and serve.

Creamy Peas

Preparation time: 10 minutes

Cooking time: 20 minutes

Servings: 4

Nutritional Values (Per Serving):

- Calories 191
- Fat 5
- Fiber 4
- Carbs 11
- Protein 9

Ingredients:

- 1 cup coconut cream
- 1 yellow onion, chopped
- 1 tablespoon olive oil
- 2 cups green peas

- A pinch of salt and black pepper
- A pinch of salt and black pepper

Directions:

1. Heat up a pan with the oil over medium heat, add the onion and sauté for 5 minutes.
2. Add the peas and the other ingredients, toss, cook over medium heat for 15 minutes, divide between plates and serve.

Purple Carrot Mix

Preparation time: 10 minutes

Cooking time: 1 hour

Servings: 5

Nutritional Values (Per Serving):

- Calories 100
- Fat 4,7
- Fiber 0,9
- Carbs 13,6
- Protein 1,2

Ingredients:

- 6 purple carrots, peeled
- A drizzle of olive oil
- 2 tablespoons sesame seeds paste

- 6 tablespoons water
- 3 tablespoons lemon juice
- 1 garlic clove, minced
- A pinch of sea salt
- Black pepper to taste
- White sesame seeds for serving

Directions:

1. Arrange the purple carrots on a lined baking sheet, sprinkle a pinch of salt, black pepper and a drizzle of oil, place in the oven at 350 degrees F and bake for 1 hour.
2. Meanwhile, in a food processor, mix sesame seeds paste with water, lemon juice, garlic, a pinch of sea salt and black pepper and pulse well.
3. Spread over the carrots, toss gently, divide between plates and sprinkle sesame seeds on top.
4. Enjoy!

Baked Potatoes and "BBQ" Lentils

Preparation time: 5 mins

Servings: 4

Nutritional Values (Per Serving):

- Calories: 140
- Fat:4 g
- Carbs:24 g
- Protein:5 g
- Sugars:606 g
- Sodium:18 mg

Ingredients:

- 2 sliced large baked potatoes
- 1 c. dry brown lentils
- 2 tsps. molasses
- 1 chopped small onion

- 2 tsps. liquid smoke
- 3 c. water
- ½ c. organic ketchup

Directions:

1. Add water, onion and lentils to the pot
2. Lock up the lid and cook on HIGH pressure for 10 minutes
3. Release the pressure naturally
4. Add ketchup, liquid smoke and molasses to the lentil
5. Sauté for 5 minutes
6. Serve over baked potatoes and enjoy!

Superb Lemon Roasted Artichokes

Preparation time: 10 mins

Servings: 2

Nutritional Values (Per Serving):

- Calories: 263
- Fat:16 g
- Carbs:8 g
- Protein:23 g
- Sugars:128 g
- Sodium:0.4 mg

Ingredients:

- 2 peeled and sliced garlic cloves
- 3 lemon pieces
- Black pepper
- 2 artichoke pieces

- 3 tbsps. olive oil
- Sea flavored vinegar

Directions:

1. Wash your artichokes well and dip them in water and cut the stem to about ½ inch long
2. Trim the thorny tips and outer leaves and rub the chokes with lemon
3. Poke garlic slivers between the choke leaves and place a trivet basket in the Instant Pot ten add artichokes
4. Lock up the lid and cook on high pressure for 7 minutes
5. Release the pressure naturally over 10 minutes
6. Transfer the artichokes to cutting board and allow them to cool then cut half lengthwise and cut the purple white center
7. Pre-heat your oven to 400 degree Fahrenheit
8. Take a bowl and mix 1 and ½ lemon and olive oil
9. Pour over the choke halves and sprinkle flavored vinegar and pepper
10. Place an iron skillet in your oven and heat it up for 5 minutes
11. Add a few teaspoon of oil and place the marinated artichoke halves in the skillet

12. Brush with lemon and olive oil mixture
13. Cut third lemon in quarter and nestle them between the halves
14. Roast for 20-25 minutes until the chokes are browned
15. Serve and enjoy!

Orange Juice Smoothie

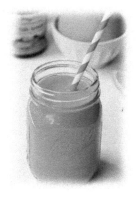

Preparation time: 5 mins

Servings: 2

Nutritional Values (Per Serving):

- Calories: 180
- Fat:0 g
- Carbs:38 g
- Protein:7 g
- Sugars:20 g
- Sodium:5 mg

Ingredients:

- ¼ c. frozen orange juice concentrate
- ¾ c. fat-free milk
- 1 c. fat-free vanilla frozen yogurt

Directions:

1. Add the Ingredients to a blender and pulse until they're smooth.
2. Pour them into frosted glasses and serve.

Chocolate Aquafaba Mousse

Preparation time: 20 mins

Servings: 4-6

Nutritional Values (Per Serving):

- Calories: 280
- Fat:13.8 g
- Carbs:34.7 g
- Protein:3.9 g
- Sugars:22 g
- Sodium:242 mg

Ingredients:

- 1 tsp. pure vanilla extract
- 15 oz. unsalted chickpeas
- Fresh raspberries
- ¼ tsp. tartar cream
- 6 oz. dairy-free dark chocolate

- 2 tbsps. coconut sugar
- ¼ tsp. sea salt

Directions:

1. Chop dark chocolate into coarse bits and place the chocolate into a glass bowl over boiling water on the stovetop or in a double boiler.
2. Melt the chocolate gently, stirring until completely melted.
3. Remove the melted chocolate from the heat and pour the chocolate into a large bowl.
4. Drain the chickpeas, reserving the brine (aquafaba), and store the chickpeas for another recipe like hummus.
5. Add in the aquafaba along with cream of tartar.
6. Mix on high speed using an electric hand mixer for 7-10 minutes, or until soft peaks begin to form.
7. Add in the salt, vanilla extract, and coconut sugar and beat the mixture until well mixed.
8. Add half of the melted chocolate to the whipped aquafaba and fold it in until incorporated.
9. Fold in the remaining aquafaba until smooth and well combined to form the mousse.

10. Gently spoon the chocolate mousse into glasses, ramekins or small mason jars.
11. Cover with cling film and chill for at least 3 hours.
12. Sprinkle he mousse with raspberries and serve.

Golden Potato Soup

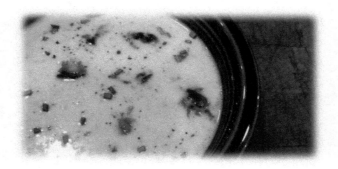

Preparation time: 5 minutes

Cooking time: 30 minutes

Servings: 4 to 6

Ingredients:

- 1 tablespoon olive oil
- 3 medium shallots, chopped
- 4 cups vegetable broth (homemade, store-bought, or water)
- 3 medium russet potatoes, peeled and diced

- 2 medium sweet potatoes, peeled and diced
- 1 cup plain unsweetened soy milk
- Salt and freshly ground black pepper
- 1 tablespoon minced chives, for garnish

Directions:

1. In large saucepan, heat the oil over medium heat. Add the shallots, cover, and cook until softened, about 5 minutes. Add the broth and potatoes and bring to a boil. Reduce heat to low and simmer, uncovered, until the potatoes are soft, about 20 minutes.

2. Puree the potato mixture in the pot with an immersion blender or in a blender or food processor, in batches if necessary, and return to the pot. Stir in the soy milk and season with salt and pepper to taste.

3. Simmer for 5 minutes to heat through and blend flavors.

4. Ladle the soup into bowls, sprinkle with chives, and serve.

Zucchini and Butter Bean Bisque

Preparation time: 5 minutes

Cooking time: 45 minutes

Servings: 4 to 6

Ingredients:

- 2 tablespoons olive oil
- 1 medium onion, chopped
- 1 garlic clove, minced
- 2 cups fresh or frozen butter beans or lima beans
- 4 cups vegetable broth (homemade, store-bought or water)
- 3 medium zucchini, cut into 1/4-inch slices
- 1/2 teaspoon dried marjoram
- Salt and freshly ground black pepper
- 1/2 cup plain unsweetened soy milk
- 2 tablespoons minced jarred pimiento

Directions:

1. In a large soup pot, heat the oil over medium heat. Add the onion and garlic, cover, and cook until softened, about 5 minutes. Add the butter beans and the broth. Cover and cook for 20 minutes. Add the zucchini, marjoram, and salt and pepper to taste. Bring to a boil, then reduce heat to low and simmer, covered, until the vegetables are soft, about 20 minutes.

2. Puree the soup in the pot with an immersion blender or in a blender or food processor, in batches if necessary, and return to the pot. Stir in the soy milk and taste, adjusting seasonings if necessary. Reheat over low heat until hot. Ladle into bowls, garnish with the pimiento, and serve.

Creamy Broccoli and Rice Bake

Preparation time: 10 Minutes

Cooking time: 40 Minutes

Servings: 7

Ingredients:

- 2 cups cooked brown rice
- 1 12-ounce bag frozen broccoli florets, chopped, or 2 cups chopped fresh broccoli florets
- ½ cup chopped onion
- 1 celery stalk, thinly sliced
- 1 batch Easy Vegan Cheese Sauce

Directions:

1. Preparing the ingredients
2. Preheat the oven to 425°F.

3. In a large bowl, mix together the rice, broccoli, onion, celery, and cheese sauce. Transfer to a 2-quart or 8-inch-square baking dish.

4. Bake for 40 minutes, or until the top has started to brown slightly.

Keto Pasta with Mediterranean Tofu balls

Preparation time: 90 minutes + overnight chilling

Serving size: 4

Nutritional Values (Per Serving):

- Calories: 232
- Total Fat:14.3g
- Saturated Fat:5.4g
- Total Carbs: 12g
- Dietary Fiber: 4g
- Sugar:4 g
- Protein:20 g
- Sodium: 719mg

Ingredients:

For the keto pasta:

- 1 cup shredded mozzarella cheese
- 1 egg yolk

For the sauce:

- 3 tbsp olive oil
- 2 yellow onions, chopped
- 6 garlic cloves, minced
- 2 tbsp unsweetened tomato paste
- 2 large tomatoes, chopped
- ¼ tsp saffron powder
- 2 cinnamon sticks
- 4 ½ cups vegetable broth
- Salt and black pepper to taste

For the Mediterranean meatballs:

- 2 cups mushroom rinds
- 1 lb tofu
- 1 egg
- ¼ cup almond milk
- 6 garlic cloves, minced
- Salt and black pepper to taste

- ½ tsp coriander powder
- ¼ tsp nutmeg powder
- 1 tbsp smoked paprika
- 1 ½ tsp fresh ginger paste
- 1 tsp cumin powder
- ½ tsp cayenne pepper
- 1 ½ tsp turmeric powder
- ½ tsp cloves powder
- 4 tbsp chopped cilantro
- 4 tbsp chopped scallions
- 4 tbsp chopped parsley
- ¼ cup almond flour
- ¼ cup olive oil
- 1 cup crumbled cottage cheese for serving

Directions:

For the pasta:

1. Pour the cheese into a medium safe-microwave bowl and melt in the microwave for 35 minutes or until melted.
2. Remove the bowl and allow cooling for 1 minute only to warm the cheese but not cool completely. Mix in the egg yolk until well combined.

3. Lay parchment paper on a flat surface, pour the cheese mixture on top and cover with another parchment paper. Using a rolling pin, flatten the dough into 1/8-inch thickness.
4. Take off the parchment paper and cut the dough into spaghetti strands. Place in a bowl and refrigerate overnight.
5. When ready to cook, bring 2 cups of water to a boil in a medium saucepan and add the pasta.
6. Cook for 40 seconds to 1 minute and then drain through a colander. Run cold water over the pasta and set aside to cool.

'or the Mediterranean tofu balls:

7. In a large pot, heat the olive oil and sauté the onions until softened, 3 minutes. Stir in the garlic and cook until fragrant, 30 seconds.
8. Stir in the tomato paste, tomatoes, saffron, and cinnamon sticks; cook for 2 minutes and then mix in the vegetable broth, salt, and black pepper. Simmer for 20 to 25 minutes while you make the tofu balls.
9. In a large bowl, mix the mushroom rinds, tofu, egg, almond milk, garlic, salt, black pepper, coriander, nutmeg powder, paprika, ginger paste, cumin powder, cayenne pepper, turmeric powder, cloves powder, cilantro,

parsley, 3 tablespoons of scallions, and almond flour.
Form 1-inch meatballs from the mixture.

10. Heat the olive oil in a large skillet and fry the tofu balls in batches until brown on all sides, 10 minutes.

11. Put the tofu balls into the sauce, coat well with the sauce and continue cooking over low heat for 5 to 10 minutes.

12. Divide the pasta onto serving plates and spoon the tofu balls with sauce on top.

13. Garnish with the cottage cheese, remaining scallions and serve warm.

SALADS

Creamy Coleslaw

Preparation time: 10 minutes

Cooking time: 0 minutes

Servings: 4

Ingredients:

- 1 small head green cabbage, finely shredded
- 1 large carrot, shredded
- ¾ cup vegan mayonnaise, homemade or store-bought
- ¼ cup soy milk
- 2 tablespoons cider vinegar
- ½ teaspoon dry mustard
- ¼ teaspoon celery seeds
- ½ teaspoon salt (optional
- Freshly ground black pepper

Directions:

1. In a large bowl, combine the cabbage and carrot and set aside.
2. In a small bowl, combine the mayonnaise, soy milk, vinegar, mustard, celery seeds, salt, and pepper to taste. Mix until smooth and well blended. Add the dressing to the slaw and mix well to combine. Taste, adjusting seasonings if necessary, and serve.

Sesame Cucumber Salad

Preparation time: 15 minutes

Cooking time: 0 minutes

Servings: 4 to 6

Ingredients:

- 2 medium English cucumbers, peeled and cut into 1/4-inch slices
- 2 tablespoons chopped fresh parsley
- 3 tablespoons toasted sesame oil
- 2 tablespoons soy sauce
- 1 tablespoon mirin
- 2 teaspoons rice vinegar
- 1 teaspoon brown sugar (optional)
- 2 tablespoons toasted sesame seeds

Directions:

1. In a small bowl, combine the cucumbers and parsley and set aside.

2. In a separate small bowl, combine the oil, soy sauce, mirin, vinegar, and sugar, stirring to blend. Pour the dressing over the cucumbers. Set aside for at least 10 minutes.

3. Spoon the cucumber salad into small bowls, sprinkle with sesame seeds, and serve.

Basil Mango Jicama Salad

Preparation time: 15 Minutes • Chill Time: 60 Minutes •
Servings: 6

Nutrition per Serving:

- Calories: 76
- Total fat: 2g
- Carbs: 14g
- Fiber: 5g
- Protein: 1g

Ingredients:

- 1 jicama, peeled and grated
- 1 mango, peeled and sliced
- ¼ cup non-dairy milk
- 2 tablespoons fresh basil, chopped
- 1 large scallion, chopped
- ⅛ teaspoon sea salt
- 1½ tablespoons tahini (optional)

- Fresh greens (for serving)
- Chopped cashews (optional, for serving)
- Cheesy Sprinkle (optional, for serving)

Directions:

1. Put the jicama in a large bowl.
2. Purée the mango in a food processor or blender, with just enough non-dairy milk to make a thick sauce.
3. Add the basil, scallions, and salt. Stir in the tahini if you want to make a thicker, creamier, and more filling sauce.
4. Pour the dressing over the jicama and marinate, covered in the fridge, for 1 hour or more to break down some of the starch. Serve over a bed of greens, topped with chopped cashews and/or Cheesy Sprinkle (if using).

Red Cabbage Slaw with Black-Vinegar Dressing

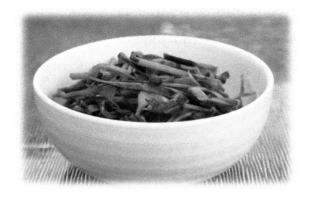

Preparation time: 15 Minutes

Cooking time: 0 Minutes

Servings: 6

Ingredients:

- 4 cups shredded red cabbage
- 2 cups thinly sliced napa cabbage
- 1 cup shredded daikon radish
- 1/4 cup fresh orange juice

- 2 tablespoons Chinese black vinegar
- 1 tablespoon soy sauce
- 1 tablespoon grapeseed oil
- 1 tablespoon toasted sesame oil
- 1 teaspoon grated fresh ginger
- 1/2 teaspoon ground Szechuan peppercorns
- 1 tablespoon black sesame seeds, for garnish

Directions:

1. In a large bowl, combine the red cabbage, napa, and daikon and set aside.
2. In a small bowl, combine the orange juice, vinegar, soy sauce, grapeseed oil, sesame oil, ginger, and peppercorns. Blend well. Pour the dressing onto the slaw, stirring to coat. Taste, adjusting seasonings if necessary. Cover and refrigerate to allow flavors to blend, about 2 hours. Sprinkle with sesame seeds and serve.

Coconut Cashew Dip

Preparation time: 10 minutes

Cooking time: 30 minutes

Servings: 4

Nutritional Values (Per Serving):

- Calories 100
- Fat 2
- Fiber 1
- Carbs 6
- Protein 6

Ingredients:

- ½ cup coconut cream
- 1 cup cashews, chopped
- 2 tablespoons cashew cheese, shredded

- 1 teaspoon balsamic vinegar
- 1 tablespoon chives, chopped
- A pinch of salt and black pepper

Directions:

1. In a pot, combine the cream with the cashew, cashew cheese and the other ingredients, stir, cook over medium heat for 30 minutes and transfer to a blender.
2. Pulse well, divide into bowls and serve.

Green Beans Dip

Preparation time: 10 minutes

Cooking time: 25 minutes

Servings: 4

Nutritional Values (Per Serving):

- Calories 172
- Fat 6
- Fiber 3
- Carbs 6
- Protein 8

Ingredients:

- 1 pound green beans, trimmed and halved
- 4 scallions, chopped
- 1 teaspoon turmeric powder
- 3 garlic cloves, minced
- 1 teaspoon rosemary, dried

- 1 and ½ cups coconut cream
- A pinch of salt and black pepper
- 1 tablespoon chives, chopped

Directions:

1. In a pan, combine the green beans with the scallions, turmeric and the other ingredients, stir, cook over medium heat for 25 minutes and transfer to a bowl.
2. Blend the mix well, divide into bowls and serve as a party dip.

Coriander Mint Chutney

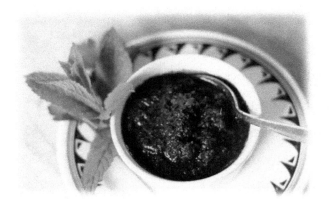

Preparation time: 10 minutes

Cooking time: 12 minutes

Servings: 4

Nutritional Values (Per Serving):

- Calories 241
- Fat 4
- Fiber 7
- Carbs 10
- Protein 6

Ingredients:

- 1 and ½ teaspoons cumin seeds
- 1 and ½ teaspoons garam masala
- ½ teaspoon mustard seeds
- 2 tablespoons avocado oil
- 2 garlic cloves, minced
- ¼ cup veggie stock
- 1 cup mint
- 1 tablespoon ginger, grated
- 2 teaspoons lime juice
- A pinch of salt and black pepper

Directions:

Heat up a pan with the oil over medium heat, add the cumin, garam masala, mustard seeds, garlic and ginger and cook for 5 minutes.

Add the mint and the other ingredients, stir, cook over medium heat for 7 minutes more, divide into bowls and serve as a snack.

Spiced Okra Bite

Preparation time: 10 minutes

Cooking time: 15 minutes

Servings: 4

Nutritional Values (Per Serving):

- Calories 200
- Fat 2
- Fiber 2
- Carbs 6
- Protein 7

Ingredients:

- 2 cups okra, sliced
- 2 tablespoons avocado oil
- ¼ teaspoon chili powder
- ¼ teaspoon mustard powder
- ¼ teaspoon garlic powder

- ¼ teaspoon onion powder
- A pinch of salt and black pepper

Directions:

1. Spread the okra on a baking sheet lined with parchment paper, add the oil and the other ingredients, toss and roast at 400 degrees F for 15 minutes.
2. Divide the okra into bowls and serve as a snack.

Rosemary Chard Dip

Preparation time: 10 minutes

Cooking time: 20 minutes

Servings: 4

Nutritional Values (Per Serving):

- Calories 200
- Fat 4
- Fiber 3
- Carbs 6
- Protein 7

Ingredients:

- 4 cups chard, chopped
- 2 cups coconut cream
- ½ cup cashews, chopped
- A pinch of salt and black pepper
- 1 teaspoon smoked paprika

- ½ teaspoon chili powder
- ¼ teaspoon mustard powder
- ½ cup cilantro, chopped

Directions:

1. In a pan, combine the chard with the cream, cashews and the other ingredients, stir, cook over medium heat for 20 minutes and transfer to a blender.
2. Pulse well, divide into bowls and serve as a party dip.

Spinach and Chard Hummus

Preparation time: 10 minutes

Cooking time: 10 minutes

Servings: 4

Nutritional Values (Per Serving):

- Calories 172
- Fat 4
- Fiber 3
- Carbs 7
- Protein 8

Ingredients:

- 2 garlic cloves, minced
- 2 cup chard leaves
- 2 cups baby spinach
- ½ cup coconut cream
- ¼ cup sesame paste

- A pinch of salt and black pepper
- 2 tablespoons olive oil
- Juice of ½ lemon

Directions:

1. Put the cream in a pan, heat it up over medium heat, add the chard, garlic and the other ingredients, stir, cook for 10 minutes, blend using an immersion blender, divide into bowls and serve.

DESSERTS

Blueberry Brownies

Preparation time: 20 Minutes

Servings: 8

Ingredients:

- 1 cup cooked black beans
- ¾ cup unbleached all-purpose flour
- ½ cup unsweetened cocoa powder
- ½ cup blueberry jam
- ½ cup natural sugar
- 1½ teaspoons baking powder
- 1 teaspoon pure vanilla extract

Directions:

1. Lightly oil a baking tray that will fit in the steamer basket of your Instant Pot.

2. Blend together the beans, cocoa, jam, sugar, and vanilla.

3. Fold in the flour and baking powder until the batter is smooth.

4. Pour the batter into your tray and put the tray in your steamer basket.

5. Pour the minimum amount of water into the base of your Instant Pot and lower the steamer basket.

6. Seal and cook on Steam for 12 minutes.

7. Release the pressure quickly and set to one side to cool a little before slicing.

Pumpkin Spice Oat Bars

Preparation time: 25 Minutes

Servings: 10

Ingredients:

- 2 cups old-fashioned rolled oats
- 1 cup non-dairy milk
- 2/3 cup canned solid-pack pumpkin
- ½ cup chopped toasted pecans
- ½ cup sweetened dried cranberries
- ½ cup packed light brown sugar or granulated natural sugar
- 6 ounces soft or silken tofu, drained and crumbled
- 2 teaspoons ground cinnamon
- 1½ teaspoons baking powder
- 1 teaspoon salt
- 1 teaspoon pure vanilla extract
- ¼ teaspoon ground nutmeg
- ¼ teaspoon ground allspice

Directions:

1. Lightly oil a baking tray that will fit in the steamer basket of your Instant Pot.
2. Stir together the oats, cinnamon, nutmeg, allspice, sugar, baking powder, and salt.
3. Blend together the tofu, pumpkin, milk, and vanilla until smooth and even.
4. Stir the wet and dry ingredients together before folding in the pecans and cranberries.
5. Pour the batter into your tray and put the tray in your steamer basket.
6. Pour the minimum amount of water into the base of your Instant Pot and lower the steamer basket.
7. Seal and cook on Steam for 12 minutes.
8. Release the pressure quickly and set to one side to cool a little before slicing.

Frutti Cobbler

Preparation time: 30 Minutes

Servings: 6

Ingredients:

- 1¼ cups unbleached all-purpose flour
- 1 cup fresh blueberries, rinsed and picked over
- 1 cup fresh blackberries, rinsed and picked over
- ¾ cup natural sugar
- ½ cup unsweetened almond milk
- 2 large ripe peaches, peeled, pitted, and sliced
- 2 ripe apricots, peeled, pitted, and sliced
- 1½ tablespoons tapioca starch or cornstarch
- 1 tablespoon vegetable oil
- 1 teaspoon baking powder
- ½ teaspoon pure vanilla extract
- ¼ teaspoon salt
- ¼ teaspoon ground cinnamon

Directions:

1. Lightly oil a baking tray that will fit in the steamer basket of your Instant Pot.
2. Toss the fruit in the tapioca and ½ a cup of sugar and put in the tray.
3. Put the tray in your steamer basket.
4. Pour the minimum amount of water into the base of your Instant Pot and lower the steamer basket.
5. Seal and cook on Steam for 12 minutes.
6. In a bowl stir together the flour, remaining sugar, cinnamon, baking powder, and salt.
7. Slowly combine with the almond milk, vanilla, and oil until soft dough is formed.
8. Release the Instant Pot's pressure quickly, give the fruit a stir, and cover with the dough.
9. Seal and Steam for another 5 minutes.
10. Release the pressure quickly and set to one side to cool a little.

Pear Mincemeat

Preparation time: 35 Minutes

Servings: 6

Ingredients:

- 4 firm ripe Bosc pears, peeled, cored, and chopped
- 1 large orange
- 1½ cups apple juice
- 1¼ cups granola of your choice
- 1 cup raisins (dark, golden, or a combination)
- 1 cup chopped dried apples, pears, or apricots, or a combination
- ½ cup packed dark brown sugar or granulated natural sugar
- ¼ cup brandy or 1 teaspoon brandy extract
- 2 tablespoons pure maple syrup or agave nectar
- 2 tablespoons cider vinegar
- ½ teaspoon ground cinnamon
- ½ teaspoon ground allspice
- ½ teaspoon ground nutmeg

- ¼ teaspoon ground cloves
- Pinch of salt

Directions:

1. Zest the orange, then peel it, deseed it, and quarter it.
2. Blend the orange flesh and zest and put in your Instant Pot.
3. Add the pears, dried fruits, juice, sugar, brandy spices, vinegar, and salt.
4. Seal and cook on Stew for 12 minutes.
5. Release the pressure naturally, take out some of the juice, then reseal and cook another 12 minutes.
6. In a bowl mix the granola and syrup.
7. Release the pressure of the Instant Pot naturally and sprinkle the crumble on top.
8. Seal the Instant Pot and cook on Stew for another 5 minutes.
9. Release the pressure naturally and serve.

Brown Betty Bananas Foster

Preparation time: 15 Minutes

Servings: 4

Ingredients:

- 6 cups cubed white bread, a little stale helps
- 4 ripe bananas, peeled and chopped
- ⅓ cup chopped toasted pecans
- ⅓ cup pure maple syrup
- ⅓ cup packed light brown sugar or granulated natural sugar
- ¼ cup unsweetened almond milk
- 2 tablespoons brandy
- ½ teaspoon ground cinnamon
- ¼ teaspoon ground nutmeg
- ¼ teaspoon ground ginger
- ⅛ teaspoon salt

Directions:

1. Lightly oil a baking tray that will fit in the steamer basket of your Instant Pot.
2. In a bowl combine almond milk, maple syrup, and the spices.
3. Roll the bread cubes in the milk mix.
4. In another bowl mix the bananas, pecans, brandy, and sugar.
5. Layer your two mixes in the tray: half bread, half banana, half bread, half banana.
6. Pour the minimum amount of water into the base of your Instant Pot and lower the steamer basket.
7. Seal and cook on Steam for 12 minutes.
8. Release the pressure quickly and set to one side to cool a little.

Bread & Butter Pudding

Preparation time: 25 Minutes

Servings: 8

Ingredients:

- 3 cups nondairy milk, warmed
- 2 cups cubed spiced bread or cake, stale is better
- 2 cups cubed whole-grain bread, stale is better
- 1 (16-ouncecan solid-pack pumpkin
- ¾ cup packed light brown sugar or granulated natural sugar
- 3 tablespoons rum or bourbon or 1 teaspoon rum extract (optional)
- 1 teaspoon pure vanilla extract
- 1½ teaspoons ground cinnamon
- ¼ teaspoon ground nutmeg
- ¼ teaspoon ground allspice
- ¼ teaspoon ground ginger
- ¼ teaspoon salt

Directions:

1. Lightly oil a baking tray that will fit in the steamer basket of your Instant Pot.
2. Put the bread cubes in the tray.
3. Mix the pumpkin, sugar, vanilla, rum, spices, and salt.
4. Slowly stir in the milk.
5. Pour the mix over the bread.
6. Pour the minimum amount of water into the base of your Instant Pot and lower the steamer basket.
7. Seal and cook on Steam for 20 minutes.
8. Release the pressure quickly and set to one side to cool a little.

Custard Bread Pudding

Preparation time: 45 Minutes

Servings: 6

Ingredients:

- 6 cups cubed white bread
- 3 cups unsweetened almond milk
- 2 cups fresh raspberries or sliced strawberries, for serving
- ½ cup vegan white chocolate chips
- ½ cup packed light brown sugar or granulated natural sugar
- ½ cup dry Marsala Pinch of salt

Directions:

1. Melt your white chocolate into a cup of the almond milk. If using your Instant Pot, keep the lid off, stir throughout.
2. Add the Marsala, sugar, and salt.
3. Clean your Instant Pot.
4. Press half the bread cubes into the insert.

5. Pour half the Marsala mix on top.

6. Repeat.

7. Seal and cook on low for 35 minutes.

8. Release the pressure naturally.

9. Serve warm with fresh berries.

Chocolate Bread Pudding

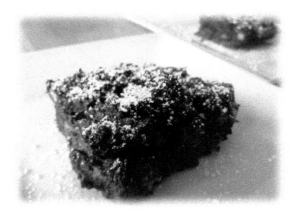

Preparation time: 40 Minutes

Servings: 6

Ingredients:

- 4 cups white bread cubes
- 2 cups unsweetened almond milk
- 2 cups vegan semisweet chocolate chips
- ½ cup chopped pecans or walnuts
- ¾ cup granulated natural sugar
- ¼ cup unsweetened cocoa powder
- 1 tablespoon vegan butter

- 1 teaspoon pure vanilla extract
- ½ teaspoon salt

Directions:

1. Oil a baking tray that will fit in your Instant Pot.
2. Melt 1 and 2/3 of the chocolate chips with 1.5 cups of the almond milk.
3. Spread the bread cubes in your Instant Pot, sprinkle with nuts, and the remaining chocolate chips.
4. Warm the remaining almond milk in another saucepan with the sugar, cocoa, vanilla, and salt.
5. Combine the cocoa mix with the chocolate chip mix and pour it over the bread.
6. Seal your Instant Pot and cook on Beans for 30 minutes.
7. Depressurize naturally.

Avocado Broccoli Soup

Preparation time: 20 minutes

Cooking time: 5 minutes

Servings: 4

Nutritions:

- Calories 269
- Fat 21.5 g
- Carbohydrates 12.8 g
- Sugar 2.1 g
- Protein 9.2 g
- Cholesterol 0 mg

Ingredients:

- 2 cups broccoli florets, chopped
- 5 cups vegetable broth

- 2 avocados, chopped
- Pepper
- Salt

Directions:

1. Cook broccoli in boiling water for 5 minutes. Drain well.
2. Add broccoli, vegetable broth, avocados, pepper, and salt to the blender and blend until smooth.
3. Stir well and serve warm.

Cauliflower Radish Salad

Preparation time: 15 minutes

Cooking time: 0 minutes

Servings: 4

Nutritions:

- Calories 58
- Fat 3.8 g
- Carbohydrates 5.6 g
- Sugar 2.1 g
- Protein 2.1 g
- Cholesterol 0 mg

Ingredients:

- 12 radishes, trimmed and chopped
- 1 tsp dried dill
- 1 tsp Dijon mustard
- 1 tbsp cider vinegar

- 1 tbsp olive oil
- 1 cup parsley, chopped
- ½ medium cauliflower head, trimmed and chopped
- ½ tsp black pepper
- ¼ tsp sea salt

Directions:

1. In a mixing bowl, combine together cauliflower, parsley, and radishes.
2. In a small bowl, whisk together olive oil, dill, mustard, vinegar, pepper, and salt.
3. Pour dressing over salad and toss well.
4. Serve immediately and enjoy.

Broccoli Casserole

Preparation time: 5 minutes

Cooking time: 30 minutes

Servings: 4

Nutritions:

- Calories: 244
- Fat: 12g
- Fiber: 3g
- Carbs: 5g
- Protein: 12g

Ingredients:

- 1 lb. broccoli florets
- 15 oz. coconut cream
- 2 eggs, whisked
- 2 cups cheddar, grated
- 1 cup parmesan, grated

- 1 tbsp. parsley; chopped
- 3 tbsp. ghee; melted
- 1 tbsp. mustard
- A pinch of salt and black pepper

Directions:

1. Grease a baking pan that fits the air fryer with the ghee and arrange the broccoli on the bottom.
2. Add the cream, mustard, salt, pepper and the eggs and toss
3. Sprinkle the cheese on top, put the pan in the air fryer and cook at 380°F for 30 minutes
4. Divide between plates and serve.

Broccoli and Almonds

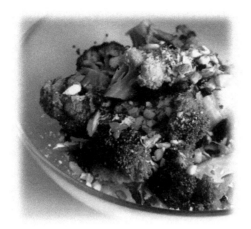

Preparation time: 5 minutes

Cooking time: 12 minutes

Servings: 4

Nutritions:

- Calories: 180
- Fat: 4g
- Fiber: 2g
- Carbs: 4g
- Protein: 6g

Ingredients:

- 1 lb. broccoli florets
- ½ cup almonds; chopped
- 3 garlic cloves; minced
- 1 tbsp. chives; chopped
- 2 tbsp. red vinegar
- 3 tbsp. coconut oil; melted
- A pinch of salt and black pepper

Directions:

1. Take a bowl and mix the broccoli with the garlic, salt, pepper, vinegar and the oil and toss.
2. Put the broccoli in your air fryer's basket and cook at 380°F for 12 minutes
3. Divide between plates and serve with almonds and chives sprinkled on top.

Rich Chickpeas and Lentils Soup

Preparation time: 10 minutes

Cooking time: 5 hours

Servings: 6

Nutritions:

- Calories 341
- Fat 5
- Fiber 8
- Carbs 19
- Protein 3

Ingredients:

- 1 yellow onion, chopped
- 1 tablespoon olive oil
- 1 tablespoon garlic, minced
- 1 teaspoon sweet paprika
- 1 teaspoon smoked paprika

- Salt and black pepper to the taste
- 1 cup red lentils
- 15 ounces canned chickpeas, drained
- 4 cups veggie stock
- 29 ounces canned tomatoes and juice

Directions:

1. In your slow cooker, mix onion with oil, garlic, sweet and smoked paprika, salt, pepper, lentils, chickpeas, stock and tomatoes, stir, cover and cook on High for 5 hours.
2. Ladle into bowls and serve hot.
3. Enjoy!

Chard and Sweet Potato Soup

Preparation time: 10 minutes

Cooking time: 8 hours

Servings: 6

Nutritions:

- Calories 312
- Fat 5
- Fiber 7
- Carbs 10
- Protein 5

Ingredients:

- 1 yellow onion, chopped
- 1 tablespoon olive oil
- 1 carrot, chopped
- 1 celery stalk, chopped
- 1 bunch Swiss chard, leaves torn

- 2 garlic cloves, minced
- 4 sweet potatoes, cubed
- 1 cup brown lentils, dried
- 6 cups veggie stock
- 1 tablespoon coconut aminos
- Salt and black pepper to the taste

Directions:

1. In your slow cooker, mix oil with onion, carrot, celery, chard, garlic, potatoes, lentils, stock, salt, pepper and aminos, stir, cover and cook on Low for 8 hours.
2. Ladle soup into bowls and serve right away.
3. Enjoy!
4. Salt and black pepper to the taste.

Lightning Source UK Ltd.
Milton Keynes UK
UKHW021404070521
383306UK00005B/94